Obamacare: A One-Line Repeal

Congress must get this done!

Despite what Democrats wanting to make Obama a modern saint will say; most thinking Americans hate Obamacare because they do not want the government in charge of their healthcare. It is that simple. Americans know that the guy who gets all the political jobs will be designated in their neighborhood as the guy who determines who gets what treatment.

Health insurance will no longer matter. Johnny B. Good, the guy who put up the spite fence next door to you—the guy with the four Pit Bulls, will cup his hands to his face after you make your plea, and then he will decide if your operation is needed. Your money won't matter when Johnny from the Neighborhood is in charge. That alone scares Americans to death.

Americans are not happy with Obamacare's increasing premium costs and its increasing share of deductibles, and they don't like that Doctors are dropping out of the program like flies giving decreasing access to professionals Americans know what they don't like. They know what they do like. They know that they do not want the government, especially neighborhood guys like Johnny B. Good making health decisions for their family. I applaud the efforts of good and honest US representatives willing to put a steel tip on their shoe and boot Obamacare out of town for good.

President Trump intrinsically knows how to do business logically without convoluted rules. The plan outlined right here in this book shows how our wonderful President can use the simplest methodology ever to repeal and replace Obamacare with a market based solution—exactly the way he promised during the campaign.

I predict that you will read this book from cover to cover in one sitting.

BRIAN W. KELLY

LETS GO PUBLISH

Title: Obamacare: A One-Line Repeal!
Copyright © November 2017,   Brian W. Kelly
Publisher: Brian P. Kelly
Author: Brian W. Kelly

Published by: LETS GO PUBLISH!
Publisher   Brian P. Kelly
Email: info@letsgopublish.com
Web site   www.letsgopublish.com

LETS GO PUBLISH

Library of Congress Copyright Information Pending
Book Cover Design by BW Kelly
Editor—Brian P. Kelly

ISBN Information: The International Standard Book Number (ISBN) is a unique machine-readable identification number, which marks any book unmistakably. The ISBN is the clear standard in the book industry. 159 countries and territories are officially ISBN members. The Official ISBN For this book is on the outside cover:

ISBN 978-1-947402-18-8

The price for this work is: $10.95 USD

10   9   8   7   6   5   4   3   2   1
Release Date: November 2017

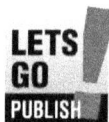

Publisher's Note: Please check out www.letsgopublish.com to read the latest version of our heartfelt acknowledgments updated for this book. On the site, please click the bottom item of the Main menu!

Dedication

Special Thanks Are Extended:

To my lovely wife, Pat,

To My Children, Brian, Michael & Katie

To My Brothers
& Sisters,

Angel Ed, Nancy Flannery, Mary Daniels & Joseph

Plus

My best buddies Dennis Grimes and Gerry Rodski.

A special dedication to Wiley Ky Eyeley!

Table of Contents

About the Author

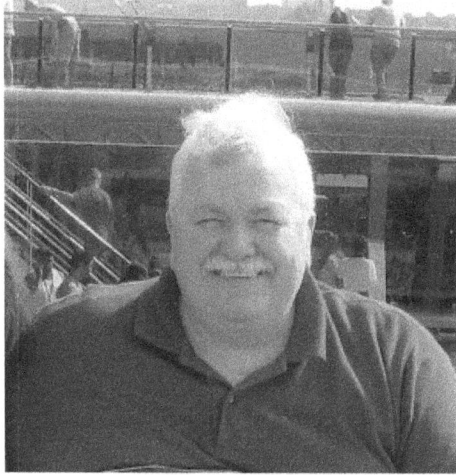

Brian W. Kelly retired as an Assistant Professor in the
Business Information Technology (BIT) program at
Marywood University, where he also served as the IBM i and
midrange systems technical advisor to the IT Faculty. Kelly
has designed, developed, and taught many college and
professional courses. He is also a contributing technical editor
to a number of IT industry magazines, including "The Four
Hundred" and "Four Hundred Guru" published by IT Jungle.

Kelly is a former IBM Senior Systems Engineer and he was a
candidate for US Congress from Pennsylvania. He has an
active information technology consultancy. He is the author
of 131 other books, in many topical areas, as well as hundreds
of articles. Kelly has been a frequent speaker at many US
conferences. Invite him to your next conference on
immigration solutions.

When Kelly ran for Congress as a Democrat against a 13-term
Democrat in 2010, he took no campaign contributions, spent
just enough to buy signs and T-shirts, and as a virtual
unknown, he captured 17% of the vote. Kelly says: "Writing
books is lots easier than running for public office!"

Chapter 1 Setting the Table

Congress is not interested in Americans or in the truth

Nobody likes a liar but unfortunately, when our friendly representatives reach Washington for the first time, they get accustomed to lies and eventually they get accustomed to lying. They smell lies wherever they go on Capitol Hill and eventually they begin to add to the stink. It is tough dealing with lies and liars in our lives. Yet, somehow, we persevere.

It would be nice if we did not have to tolerate liars such as those we send to represent our needs in Washington, But, *they say* that's how it is in politics. Our finest politicians become part of the problem as they collude with their fellow politicos to fashion common stories, which often turn out to be lies? They all know they are lying but when they give us the "facts," we are unaware that what they say, or promise, is just not the truth.

By now, we should know better; but it is tough to believe that some people are so caught up in the swamp, that they are as comfortable with fiction as they are with the truth.

After seven years of promising to repeal and replace Obamacare, the verdict is in, at least so far. When

Republicans got their chance with a majority in the Senate and the House as well as owning the presidency, they reneged. Their promise to do exactly what they said was a lie of convenience to get elected.

Let me try on what could be your next experience with Congress if you invite a Senator or Congressman to Thanksgiving dinner. Would you expect them to show even if they RSVP and tell you to expect them and their staffs?

Thank God only you and not the rest of us would be depending on Congress showing up for Thanksgiving Dinner to be a success. Their words are not too reliable. But, you invited a Senator and at least one of the most famous liars in the world agreed to come to your late November dinner fest. Clearly, for such an "honorable guest," you have no choice but to overprepare.

Depending on how many, you might go ahead and buy two extra fresh turkeys to feed them and their large entourage. They said they were coming. Time to get ready!

When Thanksgiving Dinner is ready, despite your hard work, the many extra guests are no-shows without a phone call. They are as absent from the dinner table as some of your errant, undependable family members who had promised to show but also did not.

After all your preparations for naught, you find yourself reflecting on what this means for so many to be AWOL. Were they kidding? How many others did they promise? Where did they go? Meanwhile, the two once-live Pallman Turkeys direct from the farm, that had been running around Pallman's huge barnyard, having fun and frolicking together are now cooked, stuffed, and on the table.

The two extra birds were discussing matters right before your last-minute purchase. The figured that with just a few of their buddies left, they had made the literal T-day cut. They were among the few still living and still in the Barnyard. In fact, they were convinced that they had been spared the "cut."

That was just a day earlier but now on T-day, before the long roasting, they were deader than doornails and in the home cooler, getting ready for the five-hour baking party. Why? Because a few dignitaries could not decide if they were coming or not. Death cannot be undone just because somebody lies.

Of course, there was no message saying that there would be no attendance, so your plan to roast all of the turkeys at once in the kitchen ovens plus one without stuffing in the trusty outside Turkey Fryer was designed to have everything ready when the guests arrived. But, nobody came

Yes, besides causing the unneeded death of one-time Pallman Farms turkeys, lies can also kill people. Think about those in Benghazi waiting for government help that never came. That's surely worse than the turkeys unless you are a turkey. Yet, for some reason as Thanksgiving approaches, I cannot get the Pallman hens out of my mind as a few lies surely led to their sacrifices. They were beauties and they almost made it.

So, why would or should any of us ever believe members of Congress on anything important, when they cannot come through on even the small stuff. When they promised to repeal and replace Obamacare, why did we think they were serious? Our fault for sure.

The Republican-dominated House and Senate, including War Hero John McCain during election time, promised us that we would have Obamacare repealed and replaced in 2017 and we would also have tax reform. Was the Senator kidding or lying? If he came for dinner would he have enjoyed, it?

Neither happened as the Senate led by John McCain remembered they were in Congress where all the big lies happen. Why tell the truth when a Pallman Turkey can take the axe, and nobody is the wiser? McCain put the kibosh to all hope for any action on Obamacare. And, he is still beaming proud of it.

Americans had been duped by the venerable often venerated Republicans who did not want to give up their renowned seats in the Congress. Republicans said repeal and replace Obamacare a million times while campaigning in 2016 and in fact knowing that Obama would veto their efforts, the Senate passed a repeal bill and over Obama's seven years, the House passed repeal at least 50 times before Trump promised to sign the bill if passed. Whoa! That was the end of repeal bills.

This time, the Congress's lies are more well-known than bringing on a Pallman Turkey to take the hit and then moving on to the bright side of life. Just like coming to dinner at your house or my house for Thanksgiving, the Republicans, including Maverick John McCain lied about supporting repeal and replace. It's that simple.

The press actually wrote about a Republican seven-year quest to repeal Obamacare and they offered that the whole deal ground to a halt at 1:30 AM on a particular Friday when Sen. John McCain (R-AZ) approached the podium in the Senate chamber, raised his arm, and gave the clerk thumbs down.

Obamacare repeal was, for the foreseeable future, dead. John McCain hates Donald Trump as much as he hates his own word.

The simplest explanation of why the Obamacare effort repeal failed is that McCain's vote — coupled with longstanding opposition from Sens. Lisa Murkowski (R-AK) and Susan Collins (R-ME) — meant that the Health Care Freedom Act could not move through the chamber.

Congress often uses deceit and lies to buffalo the American people. Soon, the buffaloing buffoons will be whistling their way out of their own cozy chairs as the people vote in replacement players. Americans do not like liars.

Chapter 2 Ryancare Has No Chance of Becoming Law

Silly Congressional rules must be changed

If we ever accept again a premise that Paul Ryan intends to do what is right for the American people, shame on us? Ryan claimed to put out a premise that he had constructed the best bill possible to repeal and replace Obamacare as he and the Republicans promised to the American people? There were just two things wrong with his bill: It neither repealed nor replaced Obamacare. If we can get past that, and we still think Ryan did his well-intentioned best, then he clearly failed.

If on the other hand as some suggest, Ryan's objective was to snooker the American people while snookering President Trump into thinking the only way to pass anything was to pass his elite establishment concoction euphemistically labeled as The American Healthcare Act of 2017, for a while at least, he accomplished his goal.

The bill was replete with so many twists and turns that it was as if Ryan was hoping that with enough wrong turns, it would bring him to the right place.

Unfortunately, few of us were convinced he wanted to take us anyplace good nor anyplace he had promised.

Even a duly appointed Parliamentarian would argue with another Parliamentarian about what was actually possible with the legislation. If this going the wrong way was his intention, then Paul Ryan seems to have succeeded.

The problem as we all learned but only after the bill was finally released from its top-secret chamber in the sub-basement of the House, was that the bill was a sellout. Yes, despite the Ryan-hype, the Ryancare bill, according to many who could describe it in better language, found that it stunk to high heaven. P.U.!

Nobody wanted to get close to it and nobody really wanted to touch it, and after all the work put into it; nobody wanted their name on it. The White House said not to call it "Trumpcare." Critics and Cynics began to label it alternately "Ryancare" and "Obamacare-lite." Hospitals learned to hate it in short order, and insurers began to push the panic button which automatically called all the big donors.

The House bill which Paul Ryan pushed to "repeal and replace" Obamacare quickly became a bill that nobody wanted to own. Tell me folks, do any of us think that fact alone demonstrated enough about this legislation?

 Donald Trump, God love him for his energy, was erroneously told by Mr. Ryan that what he saw, was all he could get. He was also told that Mr. Ryan as the

Speaker of the House could deliver it as it existed in a binary vote in the House. So much wanting something rather than nothing. The President went for it. He believed Ryan to be a truthful man. More and more see that supposition as a mistake!

There was a major problem causing all the stink. The bill did not accomplish the # 1 objective. It did not repeal Obamacare. How can a repeal and replace bill not do the repeal? You tell me. When Paul Ryan described the bill, many conservatives heard only "Humma humma humma" like Ralph Cramden on camera.

Great favorites of the seniors were left in the bill such as the Death Panel. Additionally, as a proportion, seniors would be the group of people that would see the most coverage losses – those aged 50 and older. How could that be? Republicans walked gingerly so that the people would not be aware the ruse was intentional.

Plus, there was no provision to get a cheaper policy across state lines or anywhere for that matter. Affordability was apparently not a concern. In essence, after the bill was examined from top to bottom, the government, not the individual, was back in control of everybody's healthcare. Who asked for that?

And, so, various people in government and the media from Rand Paul to Charles Krauthammer called it Obamacare-lite. The bill consisted of about 50% window-dressing; 35% condiments—heavy on the ketchup, and it left Obamacare's grip on the 15% meaty substance of the health of the nation. To make it look like more than it was, it also shifted some things from the right side of the page to the left, and of course when printed, it was nicely bound.

The bottom line is that it appeared hastily put together after seven years; was not well explained, and it did not solve the problem. Congress failed the American people and Congress failed Donald Trump, our President. The American people, when finally learning what it was to the extent possible, said, "NO," by a margin of 83 to 17.

The conservative sponsor of legislation to fully repeal the Affordable Care Act, aka Obamacare was Congressman Jim Jordan. He explained that the Ryan proposal was rejected by Americans because it preserved far too much of the old Obamacare system and therefore it could not be accepted. That is another way of saying that the bill simply did not repeal Obamacare.

U.S. Rep. Jim Jordan, R-Ohio is the co-founder and former chairman of the House Freedom Caucus. He had introduced legislation to fully repeal the Affordable Care Act, also known as the ACA or Obamacare. However, with Paul Ryan apparently representing the swamp faction, he knew his reasonable shot at the elimination of Obamacare would go nowhere. Ryan was fully in control and he was on a mission to subvert the people. Meanwhile there was a gag order on Republicans, so they would not bad mouth "Ryan's fine efforts." Humph! time.

Newt Gingrich said that President Trump was misled by House Speaker Paul Ryan (R-Wisc.) into believing that he could pay little attention to the Obamacare replacement bill, and come in at the end and sign it. It would be that simple for the President. It was not.

Jordan has an aversion to lying to the American people. So, he is vigorously opposed to the Ryan version of the American Health Care Act. Jordan, after examining the bill argued that it is not what Republicans had been promising voters since 2010.

"We're not repealing Obamacare. Even people who are for it, like Charles Krauthammer, have said it's Obamacare-lite," Jordan told WND and Radio America. "It keeps the Obamacare structure, and that's not what we told the voters. If you don't repeal Obamacare, you're never going to bring down the cost of insurance for middle class and working-class families."

Plus, that pesky ole death panel is still there.

"So, it is really that basic. Let's do what we said. That's what they sent us here to do. Let's actually repeal Obamacare. A clean and complete repeal is what we're after. This doesn't do it."

Few saw Ryancare as an answer to anything.

From the moment that Paul Ryan appeared as the lead spokesman for the bill, many conservatives felt it was a hose job from the start. There was nothing in it for conservatives. Normal people had been watching Ryan in action for some time as one of the major representatives of the Republican Swamp government in Washington. We'd seen him before and he came off as a bad actor. Ryan has not recovered.

There is nothing in the bill there but a bunch of spinning wheels that take the country no place. Ryan contended the plan does fulfill the promise to repeal and replace Obamacare. Yet, few people who examined the bill found very little more, if any more, than pure Obamacare

And, so, some good Americans that can read past the legalese, found that Ryan's bill does basically nothing to change the status of healthcare in the nation. Many wonder if that was Ryan's intention.

Jordan offered a number of key differences between a complete repeal and what Obamacare—lite does:

"We didn't tell voters we were going to repeal Obamacare, but we were going to keep some of the taxes in place, which the speaker's plan does. We didn't say we were going to repeal Obamacare but take the Medicaid expansion and extend it for several years, which the speaker's plan does," Jordan said. There is a lot more that Paul Ryan's bill does not do right and keeping it locked in the sub-basement of the House for months, not permitting others to view it, certainly did not help build a consensus.

Few people understand Congress because they actually give the members credit for being smart and some still think they are honest. They are foxy and very political and self-serving, for sure and they are smart in protecting their self-interests. They spend more time hiding their intentions and masking their legislation from detection than they do in writing bills that openly fulfill their promises to the people.

They use one trick after another, most of which were not in the deliberations of the founders and have no space in the Constitution. But, their tricks help them preserve their good old boy network and help reassure their reelections—their seemingly only important mission. The worst thing that we the people could ever do is say, "Well, that's just how it is in Washington?" Baloney. That's how they make it. We can't let them keep getting away with it.

In Chapter 4, I will tell you about a little trick they used recently in the Obamacare debacle to make us think that they had no control of the situation and thus, we must accept only what they choose to give us. They want us to believe that despite the fact that they run the country with Republicans as the majority, they have no way of enacting legislation on our behalf.

What can they do then if not for nothing? Why keep an expensive elite group of know-it-alls on the payroll when admittedly they cannot do anything?

There is this notion that we discuss in Chapter 4 called the Parliamentarian. Supposedly all of the balderdash fed to us by Paul Ryan was because the Senate's

Parliamentarian, who happens to be a left-over Harry Reid appointee, supposedly will stop the Senate from being able to use "reconciliation," to pass a real repeal and replace bill. In Chapter 4, I will show you why this is all claptrap. Does this mean that the 535 elected members of Congress are blaming an unelected appointee for their failures? We'll see in Chapter 4.

The point here is that all of Paul Ryan's maneuverings and in fact, outright gerrymandering is a ruse – a set up so that Americans would be prepared and willing to accept defeat on Obamacare. Thank the Lord for the patriots in the Freedom Caucus and smart people such as Jim Jordan, Ted Cruz, Mike Lee, and others.

Chapter 3 The Simple Solution

Need honest representation

I was very impressed with the work of Jim Jordan on the Obamacare repeal that I sent him a note. It included my plan that demonstrates how easy the process can be.

However, since Jordan is not my Congressman, I could not use the House Email system to reach him. I was shut-out by zip-code. I would suggest somebody in Congress offer legislation to change that as it may be convenient for Congress to receive less mail email, but it is not easier for constituents to kill trees buying paper and envelopes and having to buy postage stamps to communicate with Congress.

Anyway, if by chance, you have read any of my other books, you will have learned that I am a problem solver by trade. In IBM, my title was Senior Systems Engineer. I worked in the "field" with users of IBM's largest computer systems My contacts were chief executives, IT Managers, Programmers, and other technicians.

Systems Engineers were once an elite group in IBM and our mission was to solve problems. Sometimes they were IBM problems and sometimes they were problems that our clients were having in the use of IBM equipment. In this profession, you either got good at problem solving or you were asked to find a different profession after a year or two of no solutions,

Everybody knows how to solve a repeal and replace situation. You simply repeal and replace the item in question. It is that simple. Our Congress first decided it did not have the power to do it and then put a plan together in the form of a bill which did not accomplish the mission. That is a recipe for failure and it failed.

So, how do you get to solve a problem? Well, in brief terms, you first analyze the problem and consider alternate solutions, and then you pick a solution and make sure it can do the job. Problem solving is easy if somebody does not put artificial roadblocks such as self-made rules, and official rule interpreters such as Parliamentarians in your way.

So, I did exactly what I suggested above. It did not take long at all to have a simple solution guaranteed to work. Then I wrote it down. I put the problem statements and the solution statements together using the English language.

In my case I collected a lot of data and then looked-for information that supported my case. For example, few Americans know that only 4% of Americans are affected by Obamacare. Why all the fuss when it would actually be easy to simply cut checks from the Treasury. But it would not be fair to some.

I proceeded to write-up the analysis and the solution in a quick but crisp fashion and I submitted background information as well to my friendly local paper, The Citizens Voice.

The staff called me back in an hour or two to make sure that it was I, who had submitted the article and I affirmed it. After a few days, my family spotted my article (letter to the editor) before I had, and they told me that they liked it. When I saw it, I realized they had eliminated the front part which was the background information that made it all work. Most readers understood the formula for the solution even without the background information.

I then sent the link to the article along with the background information to my friends and family, so they would have the whole picture.

Then, I took it all and put it in a USPS envelope and mailed it to Congressman Jordan, so he would have the benefit of the simplest and easiest way to implement a repeal and replace strategy. The plan also took into consideration the fact that Obamacare could not be shut down immediately as people were still using it and depending on it.

Rather than explain it further here, let me show you first the letter I sent and then the attachments representing the simplest plan to repeal and replace

Obamacare. I hope you find it as simple and as doable as I believe it is.

March 8, 2017
Representative Jim Jordan
3121 West Elm Plaza
Lima, Ohio 45805

Dear Congressman Jordon,

Thank you for asking for the legislation promised to all Americans from Republicans regarding the complete repeal of Obamacare. I agree that what is on the table is not what was promised.

I sent a letter to my home paper, which prescribed a simple solution that Americans would like. I suspect your solution is similar. I send this to you in the event it may help. The parts that were printed in the paper are at this URL:

http://citizensvoice.com/opinion/replacing-obamacare-should-be-simple-1.2163103

The parts that were not printed show that Obamacare affects just 4% of the population. Why we are doing handstands on legislation that can be straightforward is a conundrum for me unless Washington wants to retain control of our healthcare.

The entire letter, as sent to the editor, is shown below

Brian W. Kelly

Repealing and Replacing Obamacare Should Be Simple:

First of all, the nastiest part of Obamacare is its 20,000+ pages which include the 2700 pages in the legislation and in total about 20,000 pages of regulations. US citizens need to have this onerous burden lifted from our backs.

When we consider that after 7 years, just 4% of the population is "benefiting" from Obamacare, it makes it look like a silly experiment in government buffoonery. The KISS approach should apply here (Keep It Simple, Stupid!).

Why it is taking so long to come up with a solution means government must be trying to keep control. Government should have little to no control and should make a graceful exit from running and controlling American healthcare.

Here are some facts:

Citizen population of the US is now 325 million

- 45 million get insurance from Medicare
- 70 million get insurance from Medicaid and CHIP
- 152 million get insurance from employers
- 13 million get insurance from Obamacare exchanges
- 60 million are either other-insured, self-insured or uninsured.

Under Obamacare, firms with 100 or more full-time equivalent employees (FTE) needed to insure at least 70% of their full-time workers by 2015 and 95% by 2016.

Those with 50 or less employees do not have to pay for employees' insurance. In 2015, 56% of non-elderly residents (270M *.56 = 152M) got their health insurance through work.

About 87% of the 13 million who buy Obamacare through Exchanges are getting some form of cost assistance to cover premiums and deductibles.

Costs and deductibles for those getting no subsistence are huge and unaffordable. For example, Mrs. X, a 63-year old real person recently compared prices for individual health insurance plans and can't believe what she found:

"They cost $1,200 a month, and they have a deductible of $6,000," she said. "I don't know how they think anyone can afford that." Mrs. X lives in Hull, Georgia,

Though it is only 13 million of 325 million right now who are under Obamacare, many citizens fear the government control that comes with Obamacare and its high premiums, poor access, and huge deductibles. Mrs. X will pay over $20,000 before Obamacare buys her a single aspirin.

The 87% who receive cost subsidies when surveyed, report that they are very pleased with Obamacare. This is understandable but not representative of the full population. After all, the rest of us are paying for their subsidies.

Millions like Mrs. X have realized they are too poor for Obamacare. There are lots of reasons why it is so expensive such as silly things like Mrs. X at 63 needs pre-natal care to be included in her policy. Moreover, Mrs. X can only buy insurance from somebody licensed in her state. v

The solution is very simple but just like it took 7 years for President Obama to get us to this point of crisis, it is not an overnight solution. However, with immediate action, the solution can begin immediately. I mean like tomorrow. I would project that in 2 to 2.5 years we can be 100% rid of Obamacare control of healthcare.

Here are the ingredients

1. Repeal Obamacare immediately [Use a one-line repeal] rendering the 2700 original pages of government control, with added regulations reaching 20,000 pages (three feet of paper) obsolete.

2. Begin the transition to a market-based system in two years. No citizens should be harmed during this process. The market system would have no government involvement and non-Obamacare polices, such as those from before 2010; should begin to be written immediately. The changes would include:

A. Permit insurance companies to immediately sell across state lines any policy that provides marketplace healthcare insurance to any potential subscriber. Make it so Obamacare policies may be canceled by the insured at any time during the two-year transition period if desired. No more new Obamacare policies will be issued.

B. Begin a two-year delay before all Obamacare policies are canceled. During this period, all existing healthcare insurance may stay in effect with no more than a 5% per annum increase for those that choose not to change at all. Once the move to a market solution is made by an individual or employer, the two-year hiatus for them is complete.

During the two years, the provision for children on parents' policies and the preexisting conditions stay in effect. Other good rules regarding policy cancellation also continue.

During this two-year period and no longer, the government may have to subsidize this to make up for the past ills of Obamacare. The government made a big mistake and it is proper that it pay for its mistake until the two-years is up.

C. Those who today receive subsidies for Obamacare, may keep them for the two years. Then, their cases are turned over to the states, and they may receive Medicaid if they qualify.

D. When the two-year wait is up, Medicaid control goes back to the States.

E. When Obamacare is gone in two years. these are the options: Medicare; Medicaid and Chip; Insurance from employer; Private insurance; other-insurance, self-insurance or no insurance.

Sincerely,

Brian W. Kelly

Chapter 4 Getting Stuck on Your Own Rules

When a rule does not work, logic says: remove it!

Fasting on beer for Lent is something done by Catholics and dieters alike. However, there are times that the individual modifies the rule when its benefits no longer outweigh its disadvantages. For example, when St. Patrick's Day comes as it always does right in the middle of Lent, then often a rule change (bend) is granted by the very person that made the rule.

That's the beauty of self-made rules. If they need to be changed so you won't die or, so harm does not come to you or simply because you want to make a change, you have the power. You change the rules as appropriate so that the benefits again outweigh the disadvantages.

Now, let's look at this idea called the Parliamentarian, which is a designated rule maker, one each in the House and the Senate.

The House Parliamentarian

The Parliamentarian is a nonpartisan official appointed by the Speaker of the House to render objective assistance on legislative and parliamentary procedure to the House of Representatives. During proceedings on the floor, the Parliamentarian sits to the Speaker's right on the dais.

This rule advisor is appointed by the Speaker and he or she also serves at the pleasure of the Speaker. This is a lot like at-will employment. When the Speaker no longer finds that the Parliamentarian fits his or her purpose, he may fire the person in the office and hire another. Why? The rules say so!

The current Parliamentarian is Thomas J. Wickham Jr. He succeeded John V. Sullivan (2004-2012), Charles W. Johnson III (1994–2004), William Holmes Brown (1974–1994), and Lewis Deschler (1928–1974). As you can see, prior to 1928, there was no keeper of the rules.

In other words, the house maketh the rules and the house can un-maketh the rules as they, not the rules, are elected by the people to serve.

The Senate Parliamentarian

The Parliamentarian of the United States Senate is the official advisor to the United States Senate on the interpretation of Standing Rules of the United States Senate and parliamentary procedure.

The current Parliamentarian is Elizabeth MacDonough. She is a Harry Reid appointee, who has held the office since 2012. Yes, she was appointed by the Democrats. Harry Reid was then Senate Majority Leader at the time.

MacDonough is the first female Parliamentarian and was preceded by Alan Frumin, and before that by Robert Dove, who was Parliamentarian in the mid-to-late 1990s.

The Parliamentarian is appointed by and serves at the pleasure of the Senate Majority Leader. That means Republican Mitch McConnell has the power to fire her and appoint somebody else. McConnell has the power but as upsetting as it is to constituents, the Leader is often reluctant to use his power to help the American people.

The purpose of the Parliamentarian position in the current debate is supposedly that the notion of budget reconciliation, which is how the Democrats originally passed Obamacare, is the vehicle of choice to repeal the law. But there is controversy.

Supposedly the rules say non-budget items cannot be part of the reconciliation, and the Parliamentarian may have to be consulted to find out exactly how to interpret the rules.

Therefore, regarding the use of the Parliamentarian in this issue, the House really did not need to limit 'Obamacare-lite' to avoid an imaginary Senate challenge over 'non-budgetary' items. The House itself is unconstrained by any such rules and could have passed anything it chose without being shut down by "rules."

Throughout the entire Ryancare debacle, when it surfaced in March, Paul Ryan has depicted the Senate Parliamentarian as a cruel ogre-like school teacher, eager to smack her huge yardstick across the knuckles of any Republican who dared to try to give Obamacare the full repeal and replacement treatment.

It never seemed to matter to Ryan that Republicans had promised the repeal and replace for seven years, and even went through the ordeal about 50 times. This excuse seemed to work well for Ryan as he put out a bill that he seemed to like. But, he was mostly alone as the people and some members of Congress knew Ryancare did not fulfill the promise.

Moreover, those who know Elizabeth MacDonough, the particular Parliamentarian in question, think the Ryan caricature of her is well overblown. They say that she seems more like a fair-minded judge, happy to weigh Republican arguments for why the Senate should consider broader repeal-and-replacement language under filibuster-proof reconciliation rules.

She is reported as saying that there's no reason why an Obamacare repeal bill necessarily could not have provisions repealing the health insurance regulations. Recently, as reported, Senator Mike Lee told Philip Klein, managing editor of the Washington Examiner that this Ryan subterfuge is all hokum and pure bunkum. Mike Lee reportedly discussed this matter with MacDonough on to get her perspective.

Lee is quoted as follows: "The Parliamentarian said, there's not necessarily any reason that would categorically preclude you from doing more, both on the repeal front and the replacement front. All sorts of things are possible." Lee's conversation with the Democrat-appointed Parliamentarian contradicts by a factor of at least 100% the House leadership's suggestion that MacDonough somehow had pre-analyzed the "American Health Care Act," and that its text would uproot Obamacare as far as the Senate's rules would allow.

She added that before Mike Lee took the initiative, nobody had even asked her about it. How is that? How did Ryan know if she was not consulted? Paul Ryan went through all these machinations when the Republicans have more power than ever to deep six the full Obamacare bill, which is bankrupting Americans one by one as they need health care.

For his own reasons, Paul Ryan kept using this one of the arguments consistently: "This thing is the most aggressive we can pass and can get through Senate rules." As we just learned, it is just not true." Some might call it a bold-face lie. Congress need not do a study as to why its approval rating has tanked.

Consider this. Mitch McConnell, a Republican, runs the Senate. MacDonough has a job because McConnell elected to keep her on the payroll after Reid left. The Republicans can change any rule they want with a 50% majority. This leaves us back at the question of whether Paul Ryan watered the House Bill down, so it did not meet America's needs, and then spiked it so it was never tested in the Senate.

When you are in control and you own the rulemaking process, you can make rules that help fulfill promises made. Obama is no longer in charge though it would seem otherwise.

Chapter 5   Repeal & Replace in Basement for Seven Years??

Stuck in the basement with you?

There was a big rumor that the Ryancare bill was hidden in a basement, out of view of the public, and even Senator Rand Paul could not get in to see it!

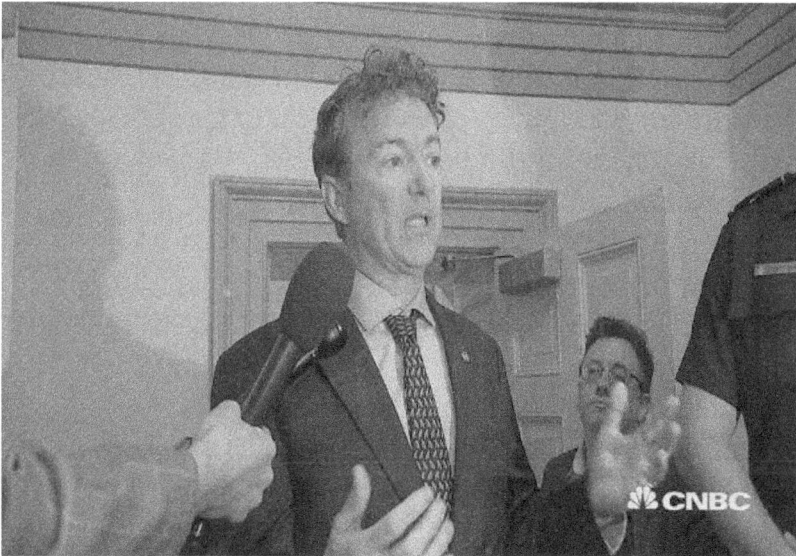

You can see in the picture that stuff like this upsets the Senator from Kentucky, who, like the general public, thinks Congress should be working for, not against the American people.

Of course, he gave it right back to the "leadership" for keeping him from seeing the bill. When we all got to see the bill, however, maybe Ryan did himself a favor by not bringing the world down upon him sooner. How could something so poorly done like this bill emerge from the basement when the Republicans had seven years to get it right?

The funny thing about it is that Paul Ryan and other members of Congress actually donned their two-peaked hats and magnifying glasses and went on a hunt to try, unsuccessfully, to get a preview of the bill. They were unsuccessful. That is not good PR for a bill that had so much riding on it.

"I have been told that the House that the Obamacare bill is under lock & key, in a secure location & not available for me or the public to view," Paul tweeted when he was about ready to hunt for it.

"This is unacceptable. This is the biggest issue before Congress and the American people right now," tweeted Paul, who has pushed for his own replacement proposal.

Paul later tweeted: "I am heading to the secure location where they are keeping the House Obamacare bill. I will demand a copy for the American people."

But those efforts went for naught, even after Paul brought along a photocopier to make his own copy of the legislation. Whose Congress is this? Whose bill is this?

"I'm not waiting until after it passes to find out what's in Obamacare, the new replacement bill." Nancy Pelosi would have advised he just sign it and find out what is in it later when he gets his own copy. You may recall that is what she did with the original Obamacare in 2010.

Paul was incensed. "This is being presented as if this were a national secret. As if this were a plot to invade another country. As if this were a national security. That's wrong. This should be done openly, in the public and conservatives who have objections who don't want Obamacare-lite should be allowed to see the bill."

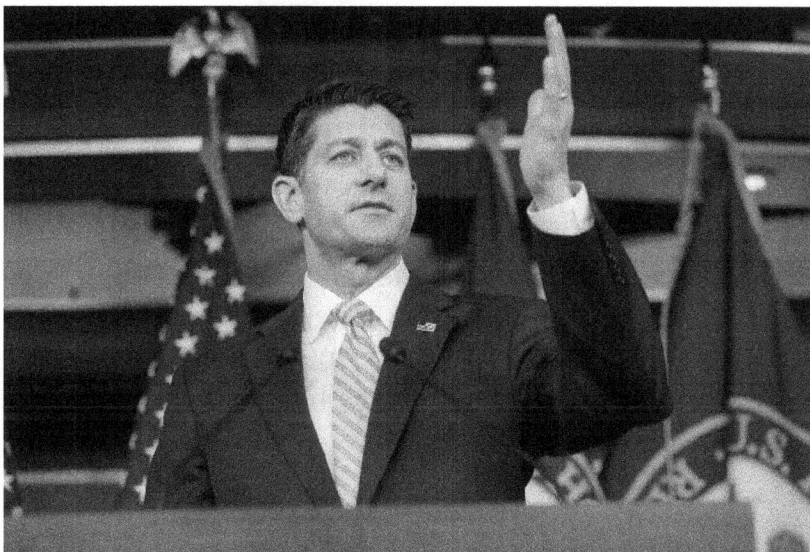

Paul Ryan stuck to his "no repeal" story. "The law is collapsing, and you can't just repeal it," Ryan said. "You have to replace it with a system that actually works." Don't you wish that Congress knew how to speak the truth.

Ryan, at the end of the briefing, was walking away from the lectern where he had been speaking, and didn't return to answer, when a reporter called out, "Why is the plan under lock and key?"

Tom Price, the Head of Health and Human Services at the time, knows a lot about a good health-care bill. The Ryan Bill is not the Price Bill. Price had introduced his Empowering Patients First Act while a Congressman representing Georgia in 2015.

His bill proposed giving every person who buys individual health insurance plans a universal tax credit, that would be adjusted by age, with older people getting more than younger people. The credits would be worth between $900 and $3,000.

Price also called for eliminating the Obamacare mandate requiring most Americans to have some form of health coverage or face a tax penalty, implement state-run high-risk pools with federal grants for people with existing health conditions, allow insurance sales across state lines, and encourage health savings accounts.

Price's bill also would repeal the expansion of Medicaid to nearly all poor adults in states that agreed to do so. Medicaid has been credited with extending health coverage to most of the 20 million Americans estimated to have become insured because of Obamacare.

The problem in all of these cherry-picking bills, is that Mr. Trump promised a full repeal, and everybody knows what a repeal is, even if Mr. Ryan has forgotten.

When Rand Paul was "looking for" the Bill, he commented: "What is the House leadership trying to hide? My guess is, they are trying to hide their "Obamacare-lite" approach.

"Renaming and keeping parts of Obamacare, new entitlements and extending Medicaid expansion are not the full repeal we promised"

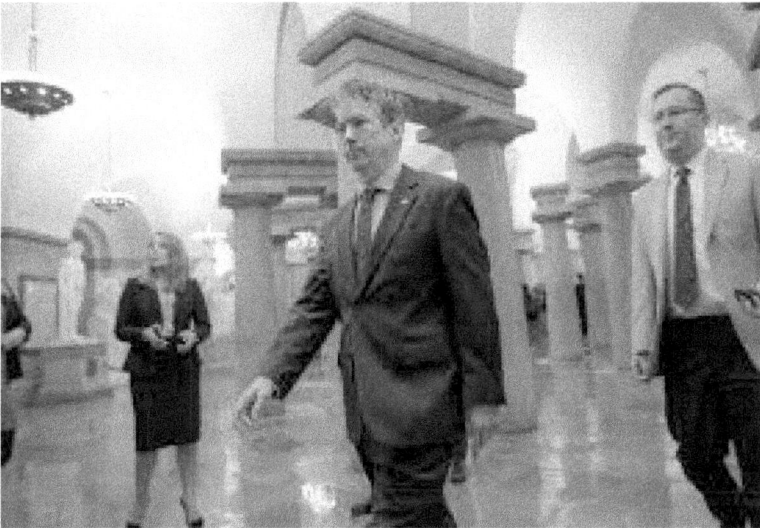

Visibly annoyed, Rand Paul noted: "I will not vote for Obamacare-lite nor will many of my colleagues. We will keep our word. I call on House leaders to do the same.

How could Paul Ryan have expected otherwise?

Chapter 6 Thank God There Is the Freedom Caucus

Nobody seems afraid of House Leadership

Many of us remember when John Boehner turned out to be a big doofus in leading the House Republicans and conservatives to any victories at all over Team Obama. Those of us not understanding the game of grab bags that was going on when Paul Ryan all-of-a-sudden wanted-in as Speaker were not very happy when it appeared that the Republicans in the House were either bought off or talked into voting for Ryan as Speaker.

You may recall that to "make it easier," Ryan immediately gave Obama all the money he needed for his agenda and that was that. We were right on Ryan.

Looks like we are right again as the on-again, off-again Trump supporter dealt the President a bad blow that Mr. Trump seems very willing to forgive. Paul Ryan is responsible for there being no Obamacare repeal and Donald Trump got himself a lesson in politics. I hope the President needs no more lessons. When you dance with the Swamp, things do not often come out as expected.

Americans, especially conservatives and nationalists are blessed with a brave Freedom Caucus in the House. Among other things, what they want is what we want—a full repeal of Obamacare. A one-line appeal is what we want.

Say it's gone in one line and permit 2700 pages of legislation to disappear along with 20,000 pages of nasty regulations. Please do not make John Q Public read each clause that is taken away to find out what is left. That will not do it and it did not do it for Paul Ryan and that is why his bill had to be pulled and it is why the Rube Goldberg version he sent to the Senate failed miserably.

Caucus Chairman Meadow, and Rep. Andy Harris gladly spoke to reporters regarding the Ryan bill. At one time, all house members were afraid to take on Paul Ryan. These two among many recognized that the Republican health-care bill, which by the time it went down in flames was known as Obamacare-lite, stood in what some called a legislative Catch-22 as late as Wednesday of the first of several decision weeks.

It had been held hostage to demands that the White House and Republican leaders claimed that they wished that they could grant but insisted that they could not. As we discussed in Chapter 4, the Parliamentarian stuff was all subterfuge and claptrap. Nobody believed it and that is why Ryan got minimal support after all the glad-handing.

The hard-liners in the House Freedom Caucus, about three dozen patriots could not move Paul Ryan to go for a real prize instead of merely changing the name from Obamacare to Obamacare-lite. Nothing Ryan did resembled a repeal option.

The whole thing would have been better managed by a combination of the Three Stooges, the Keystone Cops, and the late Steve Allen's three "men on the street." Maybe Ed Norton could have gotten a few of his co-workers in the sewer to donate some time.

Everybody has their perspective on what is right. My perspective is given in the letter I wrote to the Congressman. This is a very easy problem to solve for somebody wanting to find a solution. Give the people what we want or forever pay the political price for lying to constituents.

There is no need to even look at the eleventh-hour giveaways as the big wad of Obamacare pages was left intact in one of the poorest work products ever to come out of the House.

Donald Trump was told it was a done deal. He had to figure he could take the night off. Paul Ryan figured that he could strong-arm the House and those who did not go for that could be bribed with some kind of bonus or some legislation they liked or perhaps a committee spot for going along to get along. Don't you just hate that they bribe other Congressmen to change their minds about what is good for the people?

Ryan was asking for a vote on his health-care plan by March 23. After a day of negotiations, and after the good stubborn realists looked at surveys that said only 17% of the public was for the bill, Ryan pushed the vote back to Friday. He had to know he was not going to get what he needed but he pushed on. Ryan continued to express optimism that the bill would pass. Like many, I am so glad this bad legislation went down. Congress was playing games with the people and we are sick of it.

There are still those who want to blame the Congressional Budget and Impoundment Control CBIC Act of 1974 as the issue. We have yet to introduce this culprit into this book.

The CBIC is the federal law, passed by Congress that lays out the procedure congressional Republican leaders theoretically must use to pass the American Health Care Act — the "reconciliation" process that will ultimately allow them to pass the bill without Democratic votes.

I say theoretically because Republicans have a majority and can if they choose to, change the rules for the benefit of the people. The law as it stands dictates that not just anything can be passed by reconciliation.

For example, matters that are "extraneous" to the budgetary nature of the bill for example are excluded. However, remember that Congress can stretch a dollar into any crevice to give it a budgetary identity. Congress has so much power that if they opt to make "white" into "black," it shall be black, and vice versa.

We can bet that if there were a Congressional Bonus tied to a clean repeal, they would find a way.

House leaders, influenced strongly by the Speaker, have been consistent in insisting that any provisions rolling back the ACA's essential health benefits are indeed extraneous. Yet, as we discussed in Chapter 4, the Parliamentarian has yet to be asked and may very well have a different opinion. And, of course Mitch McConnell can write new rules.

Trying to force the Obamacare-lite down the Freedom-Caucus' throats along with the American public, Ryan argued again Wednesday of Decision Week that if the House added the necessary language to the bill, the Senate couldn't just strip it out — it could no longer consider it as a privileged reconciliation bill needing only a simple, Republican majority to pass.

I am sorry folks, I may be nobody, but I am not buying that. When you are in control of the rules, you win if you want to. If you don't want to win, you get to use the opponents' interpretation of the rules.

Ryan believed he would bowl over the house because of his power position but he could not.

"Look, our whole thing is we don't want to load up our bill in such a way that it doesn't even get considered in the Senate," Ryan told radio host Hugh Hewitt on Wednesday morning.

"Then we've lost our one chance with this one tool we have, reconciliation. It doesn't last long. But if the

Senate can add things to the bill, then we're all for that."

Still speaking doubletalk on something that should be clear makes it doubtful that you and I can ever win this battle with entrenched establishment elites from the SWAMP. They do not seem to be on our side.

I regret to say that White House bought a lot of the Ryan arguments and defended the troubled health-care bill a bit too vigorously. It would have died sooner as it should have if President Trump and his coterie had given it the short shrift.

The White House was not interested in anything that looked like a defeat, but Ryan had stacked the deck so that a victory was a defeat.

Ryan and White House officials — including Vice President Pence offered the Freedom Caucus a bona fide commitment that the Senate would seek to add a repeal of the essential Obamacare health benefits to the House bill once it arrived in that chamber.

The deal was that if at that point, the Senate Parliamentarian ruled that the provision(s) was / were extraneous, the good stuff needed by the people and President Trump to keep his promise would simply be dropped from consideration and removed while the rest of the bill, AKA, Obamacare-lite would remain.

Sorry, Mr. Ryan, not good enough for Americans!

Everybody was squirming trying to fit Ryan's square peg in a round hole while Americans at 83 to 17 saw it for what it was, a square peg that would not fit into a round hole.

Why would a group such as the Freedom Caucus take on faith something that otherwise they would control? So, they flatly did not accept the argument that it would be procedurally fatal to the legislation. Who cares if bad legislation was prevented from passing?

As we discussed in Chapter 4, the hokum and pure bunkum associated with all of this is because Paul Ryan tried to get intelligent human beings to believe that the decision on what is permissible in a reconciliation bill — and what House provisions would be fatal — lies in the hands of the Senate Parliamentarian, an unelected Harry Reid appointee, Elizabeth MacDonough. Come on Noah, do we need another flood to open their eyes?

Ted Cruz, still fighting for America after recovering from his own personal sting has put out an argument, that even if MacDonough were to rule against repealing the insurance mandates, she could be overruled by Pence, who is the President of the Senate.

Don't they have a lot of tricks they can use on something that simply ought to be proposed as I suggested in Chapter 3, and voted on – up or down. And, those Republicans and Democrats who would vote against the right legislation, as the old Irish balladeer once said, "We will know them by their limp!"

Senate leaders, holding on to all their personal power meanwhile, did not like the idea that the VP could come out of the darkness into the light to be the hero of the day. They dismissed the idea that the VP, the highest-ranking member of the Senate could unilaterally decide to override the Senate budget rules. Really! And who says so? And, why?

Roy Blunt was one of the Scared-E-Cats who was worried the courts would get the issue and then we would have a Constitutional Crisis. I would say we have a Constitutional Crisis already and that Congress plus President = 2, and the Judiciary is just 1. Two beats one any day of the week and that is it.

"The Vice President, and even 51 Senators without the Vice President, can't decide what the law says," Blunt said. "If you want to for sure to wind up in court, the way to do it is to decide that we've redefined the law."

Conservatives could promise to ignore that law, he added, but doing so would only lead to disappointment: "It is always a mistake to try to convince people do something you can't possibly do."

Mr. Blunt, you should know after so many deaths that "Cowards die many times before their death. The valiant never taste of death but once."

The will of the people—not a few people in black robes shall always prevail. That's how our country was designed, and I am so happy we have our wonderful Constitution.

Chapter 7 Are Only Hardnosed Conservatives and Nationalists Trying to Save America?

Who Should Americans Believe?

One of the country's finest spokespersons on matters that affect the people of the land, Louie Gohmert appeared on FOX & Friends on "must-pass" Friday morning with Clayton Morris.

President Trump will never die a coward's death as he is as brave as it comes and on this particular Friday, he brought his tweet machine out early.

President Trump's tweet on this day was strategic in that it attempted to put conservatives into a corner in order to get Paul Ryan's Anti-Trump health care bill passed.

Congressman Louie Gohmert can always be counted on for help for the people, and on this bill, Obamacare-lite, we needed his help immensely.

Gohmert said that House GOP leadership (Spelled R-Y-A-N) had "lied to the president" about not being able to fully repeal Obamacare through the budget reconciliation process in the Senate because of the so-called "Byrd rule."

Finally, we hear some truth even though it exposes a lie that I thought from moment one that it was a big lie sent directly from the people in the swamp.

Congressman Gohmert said that because the American Health Care Act or AHCA (aka: Obamacare 2.0, RINOCARE, Ryancare, Trumpcare, Swampcare, or Obamacare-lite), keeps in place the full punishing Obamacare apparatus, there would be nothing to stop a future Democrat administration from restarting Obamacare fully with little effort.

The esteemed Congressman also noted that with Obamacare-lite, health care insurance premiums would continue to unnecessarily skyrocket. Yes, you may call it the **Ryan and Trump** bill, but we should differentiate the snookerer from the snookeree.

I hated to see Mr. Trump fall into the Swamp when he thought he had enlisted a good and truthful ally. Republican leadership has been absent all during the Obama years and now with the Trump haters, it is even tougher to find the truth in their haystack

What is there to not get her folks? Americans are not stupid though Paul Ryan has played us for stooges since his appointment as the Speaker. He may even be worse than Boehner who always sweated and cried alligator tears when he was lying. At least we knew! Gohmert offered: "It [AHCA] isn't going to work. We're told that the prices [of insurance premiums] will probably go up 75% or so but maybe in the third year they may come down 10%."

"We're told that we should be thrilled that we're going to give so much more power to the federal government — to Health and Human Services — under our bill and they [House GOP leadership] don't have an answer for what it's all about when it's a Democrat in charge and not a Republican."

Louie Gohmert tells it like it is. The fake repeal bill is built on a "false premise," Gohmert said, noting that they "lied to the president" about the "thread the needle" excuse that everything must be done in the bill according to the Senate Parliamentarian's wishes. It is simply not true.

Has Paul Ryan recently attended either an MSM class or a Democrat propaganda seminar because he has gotten good at shoveling their spew.

What does Ted Cruz say about it?

The onlookers suggest that constitutional conservative Ted Cruz shredded RINO Paul Ryan on the Obamacare-lite bill. It's a deceptive and dishonest claim that Obamacare can only be repealed under three phases and Cruz avers that the "repeal and replace" bill known as the American Health Care Act (AHCA) only repeals two of the 12 free market-killing mandates of Obamacare that have made insurance premiums unnecessarily skyrocket.

Why would Paul Ryan not have told Donald Trump that and why would he not have told that to the American people?

Cruz was on TV Sunday of decision week on liberal stations as Fox had the lying big guns on their station. Cruz appeared Sunday on CBS's Face the Nation with host John Dickerson, the Texas Senator always says what he thinks.

This time, he said that he will not vote for a bill that does not lower healthcare insurance premiums and that if Republicans offer up a bill that causes premiums to continue to spiral out of control, voters "will tar and feather" them "in the streets" and it would be justified.

"I've got to tell you, if Republicans hold a big press conference and pat ourselves on the back that we've repealed Obamacare and everyone's premiums keep going up, people will be ready to tar and feather us in the streets, and quite rightly," Cruz told Dickerson, noting that the bill as written would not pass in the U.S. Senate where Republican hold a slim two-vote majority.

Cruz made the case that anyone who believes in the so-called "three-bucket solution" with all the goodies in step three is being suckered because it takes eight Democrats and now you can't get eight Senate Democrats to agree on even saying the words "good morning."

Besides eating all they can and wanting more, rats will abandon a sinking ship if they are convinced they are in peril. It is not their favorite option, however. They'd rather talk the Captain into taking the sinking lug onto the shore, where their little furrinesses may not even have to get wet.

And for those wondering how Paul Ryan has lasted so long in the House when his own people do not particularly like him, remember this. Rats cans swim.

Chapter 8 A Kind Message for President Trump & Congress

Writing a speech or presentation – three properties

When giving a speech and even when writing a paper or a book, nobody in the audience knows the subject material better than the speaker or the writer. And, so, teachers of prose and of speech advise students when writing to include these use three main ideas.

For example, here's what Dale Carnegie had to say about how to start a speech and keep audiences engaged: "Tell the audience what you're going to say, say it; then tell them what you've said."

So, now as we are closing in on all that needs to be said in this book, I will use the Carnegie method with some modifications to set the stage for the close of this book.

We have spent about sixty pages or so discussing something that could have been repealed in one line. Obamacare will not be around long for sure as it is decaying and creating more issues in America today than it is solving.

We took for granted in the beginning of the book that most Americans want the 2700-page legislation repealed along with the 20,000 pages of regulations. The 2700 pages plus 20,000 pages are available for anybody who wants to read them. And, so we spent no time explaining what is in the huge bill and subsequent regulations.

Our intention was to show how easy a Congress wishing to repeal and replace Obamacare could accomplish its mission. We talked turkey in Chapter 1 and accomplished most of the mission in Chapter 3.

We then went through a number of chapters in which we unmasked the excuses for why Obamacare could not be repealed and replaced rather than create another legislative folly. From here we scoured the news and found a number of different positions on the how's of getting the job done.

We looked at Speaker Ryan's supposed constraints and we looked at the Freedom Caucus and its positions, and then we found some prominent Congressional Figures such as Louis Gohmert and Ted Cruz and Mike Lee, so we had a rounded perspective of views on the matter. All the while, of course I have been injecting my own views which of course place Congress in an unfavorable light for trying very hard not to do its job well.

So, now, here we are in the wrap-up section of the book. Since the original proposition of repeal and replace and delay a few years to finish off Obamacare once and for all, and since nobody knows my recommendation better than I, as my summary of how to do the one-liner, I will use the same arguments from

Chapter 3 about the correct way to get this job done with the smallest amount of pain. Then next chapter, I offer an exhortation to Congress and the President about never trying to sneak anything like this down the throats of the American Public ever again.

Send the first message, first!

First, let's provide a repetition of the simple proposition that repealing Obamacare should not be difficult. After all, it is an abomination. Why should anybody have to explain themselves.

So that you don't have to roll back any pages, here it is exactly from the front of the book in Chapter 3:

Repealing and Replacing Obamacare Should Be Simple:

First of all, the nastiest part of Obamacare is its 20,000+ pages which include the 2700 pages in the legislation and in total about 20,000 pages of regulations. US citizens need to have this onerous burden lifted from our backs.

When we consider that after 7 years, just 4% of the population is "benefiting" from Obamacare, it makes it look like a silly experiment in government buffoonery. The KISS approach should apply here (Keep It Simple, Stupid!).

Why it is taking so long to come up with a solution means government must be trying to keep control. Government should have little to no control and should make a graceful exit from running and controlling American healthcare.

Here are some facts:

Citizen population of the US is now 325 million

- 45 million get insurance from Medicare
- 70 million get insurance from Medicaid and CHIP
- 152 million get insurance from employers
- 13 million get insurance from Obamacare exchanges
- 60 million are either other-insured, self-insured or uninsured.

Under Obamacare, firms with 100 or more full-time equivalent employees (FTE) needed to insure at least 70% of their full-time workers by 2015 and 95% by 2016.

Those with 50 or less employees do not have to pay for employees' insurance. In 2015, 56% of non-elderly residents (270M *.56 = 152M) got their health insurance through work.

About 87% of the 13 million who buy Obamacare through Exchanges are getting some form of cost assistance to cover premiums and deductibles.

Costs and deductibles for those getting no subsistence are huge and unaffordable. For example, Mrs. X, a 63-year old real person recently compared prices for individual health insurance plans and can't believe what she found:

"They cost $1,200 a month, and they have a deductible of $6,000," she said. "I don't know how they think anyone can afford that." Mrs. X lives in Hull, Georgia,

Though it is only 13 million of 325 million right now who are under Obamacare, many citizens fear the government control that comes with Obamacare and its high premiums, poor access, and huge deductibles. Mrs. X will pay over $20,000 before Obamacare buys her a single aspirin.

The 87% who receive cost subsidies when surveyed, report that they are very pleased with Obamacare. This is understandable but not representative of the full population. After all, the rest of us are paying for their subsidies.

Millions like Mrs. X have realized they are too poor for Obamacare. There are lots of reasons why it is so expensive such as silly things like Mrs. X at 63 needs pre-natal care to be included in her policy. Moreover, Mrs. X can only buy insurance from somebody licensed in her state. v

The solution is very simple but just like it took 7 years for President Obama to get us to this point of crisis, it is not an overnight solution. However, with immediate action, the solution can begin immediately. I mean like tomorrow. I would project that in 2 to 2.5 years we can be 100% rid of Obamacare control of healthcare.

Here are the ingredients

1. Repeal Obamacare immediately [Use a one-line repeal] rendering the 2700 original pages of government control, with added regulations reaching 20,000 pages (three feet of paper) obsolete.

2. Begin the transition to a market-based system in two years. No citizens should be harmed during this process. The market system would have no government involvement and non-Obamacare polices, such as those from before 2010; should begin to be written immediately. The changes would include:

A. Permit insurance companies to immediately sell across state lines any policy that provides marketplace healthcare insurance to any potential subscriber. Make it so Obamacare policies may be canceled by the insured at any time during the two-year transition period if desired. No more new Obamacare policies will be issued.

B. Begin a two-year delay before all Obamacare policies are canceled. During this period, all existing healthcare insurance may stay in effect with no more than a 5% per annum increase for those that choose not to change at all. Once the move to a market solution is made by an individual or employer, the two-year hiatus for them is complete.

During the two years, the provision for children on parents' policies and the preexisting conditions stay in effect. Other good rules regarding policy cancellation also continue.

During this two-year period and no longer, the government may have to subsidize this to make up for the past ills of Obamacare. The government made a big mistake and it is proper that it pay for its mistake until the two-years is up.

C. Those who today receive subsidies for Obamacare, may keep them for the two years. Then, their cases are turned over to the states, and they may receive Medicaid if they qualify.

D. When the two-year wait is up, Medicaid control goes back to the States.

E. When Obamacare is gone in two years. these are the options: Medicare; Medicaid and Chip; Insurance from employer; Private insurance; other-insurance, self-insurance or no insurance.

Chapter 9 Final Message to the President & Congress

Who knows what good lurks in the hearts of men?

I am signing off this book with another letter which I wrote to a second Paper in my home town—The Times Leader. Many of us were concerned for a short while at least that our President, with whom we are so pleased, may have begun to take his cues from the swamp. It is the same swamp he had promised to drain. We got a bit heartsick, but we recovered.

We want only what is best for President Trump as the top official of our country. We support our President 100% and we are looking for many successes to help make America great again. We are all eager to see the goodness come. We can handle it. We love winning.

As the eponymous group Phish often sang at their concerts, "Maybe So, Maybe Not!' Some were thinking Maybe Trump is for the people and maybe not. Maybe Trump is for the people and he was lied to and snookered. My hope is that the latter is true, and a much bigger Donald Trump will emerge, who does not have to win all the time but who can win victories, big or small for the people of America.

I was very disappointed in what was happening while Paul Ryan was ramming Obamacare-lite. I wanted Trump to treat Ryan like he treated Bob Corker and Jeff Flake, prompting them not to run again for the Senate. I was ready to blame my man, my hero, my guy—a man whom I had defended to the corners of the earth.

I still loved Donald Trump 8 to 20 million times more than the lying, anti-American Obama, but I desired so much for Mr. Trump to be 99 44/100% pure, I worried when he was not. So, in desperation, I wrote another editorial piece to the local paper. I hoped Mr. Trump would read it and know that sometimes he needs to give us a fireside chat to restore our faith.

This time I picked the Times Leader as I am pushing my luck when I try to get two pieces published in less than a month in the same local newspaper. I have gotten over my pain. We all learned during the Ryan ordeal and I hope the lesson sticks.

I am for Donald Trump for sure and I would like Donald Trump to do more for himself by helping us when he can to understand what he is doing and why he is doing it. That would have helped me.

Mr. Trump, please keep up the fine work and don't be so trusting when dealing with the Swamp people.

Here is the short essay:

A promise is a promise; A repeal is a repeal

"My conservative friends feel betrayed by the Republican Establishment. Why should they not? As I look at their rationale, they have good reason to feel betrayed with the new Obamacare-lite. We all do. When running for President, Donald Trump made a few promises about Obamacare. Remember this:

"On Day One, repeal Obamacare and replace it with something terrific!" Now, President Trump says he is "proud" to support a GOP-authored plan to replace Obamacare (What happened to repeal?) and he told the GOP leaders behind closed doors that he would support it "100%," according to sources in the room. This will signify the end of trust for the Trump Administration.

There is one big problem with this. Republicans, who most conservatives do not trust at all, in my opinion, and I have no reason to think otherwise, have no plan to ever repeal the 2700 pages of legislation and 20,000 pages of regulations in Obamacare.

They lied to get elected as they lied when they needed the House and then the Senate to "get things done," and then they said that was not enough.

Now, they have the presidency and they are lying again. They have no plans to repeal Obamacare. Day 1 is long past! The GOP plan merely takes government control of healthcare from the Democrats and turns it over to Republicans. Conservatives want the government out of the healthcare business—period. A one-line repeal would have been all the work they needed to do. What part of the word "repeal" do Republicans not understand?

A promise is a promise. Will this promise echo for years like another: "You can keep your policy... you can keep your doctor?

Dear President Trump. Your constituents, loyal as sin for sure believe that a repeal is a repeal. Mr. Trump, I hope that you do not take the good will of the American people for granted. There is no reason to create any doubt in our hearts about the fervor, which we displayed when we backed you, and you alone. Please get to know us.

Amen!

P.S.

I am not sure where this is going to take us, but it is not a good sign that the President now wants to battle conservatives. This is very disheartening:

From the Washington Post March 30, 2017:
President Trump effectively declared war Thursday on the House Freedom Caucus, the powerful group of hard-line conservative Republicans who blocked the health-care bill, vowing to "fight them" in the 2018 midterm elections.

In a morning tweet, Trump warned that the Freedom Caucus would "hurt the entire Republican agenda if they don't get on the team, & fast." He grouped its members, all of them Republican, with Democrats in calling for their political defeat — an extraordinary incitement of intraparty combat from a sitting president.

This is not good!

Find out what happened over the Spring and Summer in the next chapter

Chapter 10 US Senate Rejects Everything but Obamacare Itself

Eventually, the House barely passed a later version of Paul Ryan's Obamacare-Lite with the President's urging, the bill itself almost got arrested by the Parliamentarian in the Senate for malingering. It was going nowhere fast.

Months passed by with one promise after another but no resolve by Senators to do anything that moved the ball forward. Finally, after a bunch of defeats, Obamacare Lite after various concoctions, died an ignominious death on July 28 after some drama orchestrated by John McCain and two other RINO Senators.

In Ryancare's last Senate gasp, on July 28, the three GOP Senators joined their Democrat buddies to vote against a so-called skinny repeal bill, an 11th-hour effort to keep the health-care debate alive despite Republicans admitting it really was a "fraud" and a "disaster."

It was John McCain, whose hatred for President Trump becomes more and more apparent each time he appears in public, who unexpectedly killed the legislation after 1:30 A.M. on that Friday. This concluding an unprecedented multi-day legislative drive in the Senate. A few hundred protesters, keeping a vigil, cheered outside the Capitol as word reached them that it was over. Obamacare was alive, and it seemed that it would stay alive thanks to Gentleman John McCain—the Maverick.

Finishing off their August recess after taking it on the chin from the constituents at home, the Republicans quickly cobbled together another bill known as Graham-Cassidy from its two sponsors. Both Cassidy and Graham were on the talk-show circuit to convince us all that this was a better deal that a one-line repeal. It did not sway me as I think the Senate ought to keep its promises.

Trying to avoid another John McCain Maverick Victory Lap complete with a-big-thumbs down, on September 26, Republicans admitted they could not get the job done for Americans and they punted. Nobody has been found yet claiming to have received the punt.

McConnell knew Graham Cassidy would be defeated if he permitted a vote. The Leader said that he would not bring the Graham-Cassidy bill — the latest GOP repeal bill, to the floor for a vote, though it had gained steam in September after the rest break.

The tattered folder for all the bills was suffering from a malingerer's disease and it checked itself into a clinic where today it is being ministered for the disease. Rumor has it that it may be back again as the ruse of Obamacare repeal and replace continues.

As expected, if the bill were voted upon, it was doomed. Every Senate Democrat opposed the bill. Some are beginning to believe Democrats work for Vladimir Putin full-time and that explains his interest in our elections. Additionally, three Senate Republicans — Rand Paul (KY), John McCain (AZ), and Susan Collins (ME), three blokes who Putin refused to hire, — were negative and this was enough to ensure that the bill was headed for defeat.

It is going to be tough enough for Senators to get reelected so rather than force vulnerable senators to take another politically damaging vote certain to end in failure, McConnell chose not to hold the vote at all.

"We don't have the votes," Sen. Bill Cassidy (R-LA), a co-author of the bill, said at a press conference... And since we don't have the votes, we will postpone that vote."

Sen. Lindsey Graham (R-SC), the other co-author, was publicly optimistic and asserted that his bill would pass eventually. "We're coming back to this after taxes."

We'll see!

What do the people want?

A one-line repeal bill is all that is needed and then let the Marketplace takeover with a few well-meaning tweaks if necessary. But, just a few!

I am not the first to suggest a very short bill. But, I am the first to suggest a one-line bill.

On March 28, 2017 as reported by Fox News, an Alabama congressman introduced a one-sentence bill in the House Friday to repeal Obamacare. I love that my recommended bill size is smaller, but I am more tickled that there are others that think the charade of repeal and replace has gone on too long. Just repeal.

Let the marketplace replace it!

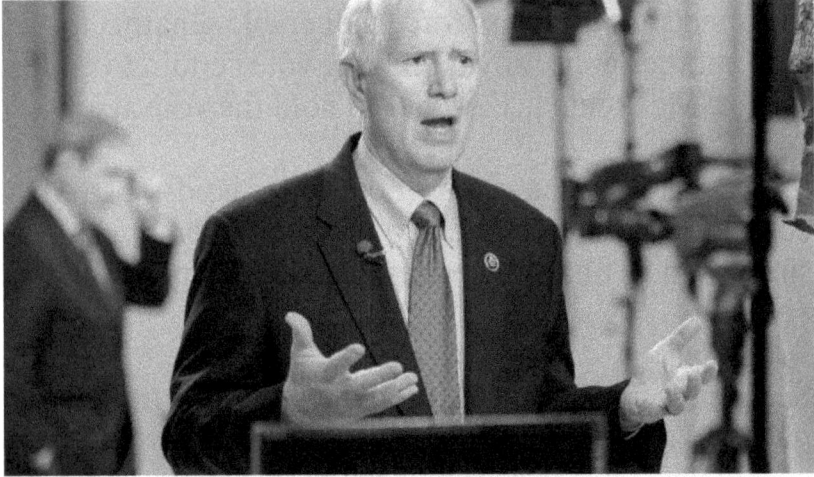

Mo Brooks has become one of my living heroes

Republican Representative Mo Brooks from Alabama, introduced the bill as the Obamacare Repeal Act.

AL.com reported the big sentence:

"Effective as of Dec. 31, 2017, the Patient Protection and Affordable Care Act is repealed, and the provisions of law amended or repealed by such Act are restored or revived as if such Act had not been enacted," The following text would be my one-line repeal:

Obamacare repealed immediately. Specifics to follow.

Don't you just love the tone?

Brooks introduced the bill after he announced that he was against Ryancare, which in its early incarnation, was pulled from a House floor vote because it did not have enough support to pass.

"If the American people want to repeal Obamacare, this is their last, best chance during the 115th Congress," Brooks said in a statement. Those Congressmen who are sincere about repealing Obamacare may prove it by signing the discharge petition…"

"At a minimum, the discharge petition will, like the sun burning away the fog, show American voters who really wants to repeal Obamacare and who merely acts that way during election time."

The bill was not voted on as Paul Ryan considered it a symbolic gesture. Isn't that reflective of why there is little trust in our Congress, especially its leadership.

Mo Brooks constructed and presented a great bill which would not have been a symbolic gesture if Congress wanted to assure that it kept its promise to repeal and replace Obamacare. They could have passed it.

The replace part was implicit as once Obamacare was repealed, insurance companies from all over the world would be flocking like buzzards to the US with the most innovative policies you have ever seen since the beginning of Obamacare.

By the way, though I like my one-line repeal, I would go with Mo Brooks one sentence repeal as it does the same thing.

Other books by Brian Kelly: (amazon.com, and Kindle)

LETS GO PUBLISH! Books by Brian W. Kelly
(Sold at Amazon.com, and Kindle.).

Obamacare: A One-Line Repeal Congress must get this done.
A Wilkes-Barre Christmas Story A wonderful town makes Christmas all the better
A Boy, A Bike, A Train, and a Christmas Miracle A Christmas story that will melt your heart
Pay-to-Go   America-First Immigration Fix
Legalizing Illegal Aliens Via Resident Visas Americans-first plan saves $Trillions. Learn how!
60 Million Illegal Aliens in America!!! A simple, America-first solution.
The Bill of Rights By Founder James Madison Refresh *your knowledge of the specific rights for all*
Great Players in Army Football Great Army Football played by great players..
Great Coaches in Army Football Army's coaches are all great.
Great Moments in Army Football Army Football at its best.
Great Moments in Florida Gators Football Gators Football from the start. This is the book.
Great Moments in Clemson Football CU Football at its best. This is the book.
Great Moments in Florida Gators Football Gators Football from the start. This is the book.
The Constitution Companion. A Guide to Reading and Comprehending the Constitution
The Constitution by Hamilton, Jefferson, & Madison – Big type and in English
PATERNO: The Dark Days After Win # 409. Sky began to fall within days of win # 409.
JoePa 409 Victories: Say No More! Winningest Division I-A football coach ever
American College Football: The Beginning From before day one football was played.
Great Coaches in Alabama Football Challenging the coaches of every other program!
Great Coaches in Penn State Football the Best Coaches in PSU's football program
Great Players in Penn State Football The best players in PSU's football program
Great Players in Notre Dame Football The best players in ND's football program
Great Coaches in Notre Dame Football The best coaches in any football program
Great Players in Alabama Football from Quarterbacks to offensive Linemen Greats!
Great Moments in Alabama Football AU Football from the start. This is the book.
Great Moments in Penn State Football PSU Football, start--games, coaches, players.
Great Moments in Notre Dame Football ND Football, start, games, coaches, players
Cross Country With the Parents A great trip from East Coast to West with the kids
Seniors, Social Security & the Minimum Wage. Things seniors need to know.
How to Write Your First Book and Publish It with CreateSpace
The US Immigration Fix--It's all in here. Finally, an answer.
I had a Dream IBM Could be #1 Again The title is self-explanatory
WineDiets.Com Presents The Wine Diet Learn how to lose weight while having fun.
Wilkes-Barre, PA; Return to Glory Wilkes-Barre City's return to glory
Geoffrey Parsons' Epoch... The Land of Fair Play Better than the original.
The Bill of Rights 4 Dummmies! This is the best book to learn about your rights.
Sol Bloom's Epoch ...Story of the Constitution The best book to learn the Constitution
America 4 Dummmies! All Americans should read to learn about this great country.
The Electoral College 4 Dummmies! How does it really work?
The All-Everything Machine Story about IBM's finest computer server.

Brian has written 132 books in total. Other books can be found at amazon.com/author/brianwkelly

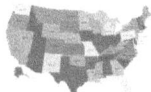

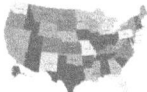

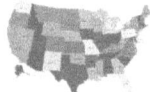

www.ingramcontent.com/pod-product-compliance
Lightning Source LLC
Chambersburg PA
CBHW071235200326
41521CB00009B/1492